How To Make Your First BDSM Scene Amazing

for Dominant Women

'How To' Femdom Series

Sharyn Ferns

How To Make Your First BDSM Scene Amazing: For Dominant
Women / Sharyn Ferns -- 1st ed.
ISBN-10: 1984068016
ISBN-13: 978-1984068019

This book is part of the 'How To' Femdom Series.

Cover art by the incredibly talented Submissive Guy Comics:
http://submissiveguycomics.tumblr.com/

Author website:
https://www.domme-chronicles.com

To new dominant women:
You are amazing and strong.
Get out there and have some fucking fun!

Table of Contents

INTRODUCTION

This is one of a series of short, sharp 'How To' Femdom guides designed for new dominant women and submissive men who want to get their hands on practical information from someone with experience.

This series of books contains tips, practical steps, and examples for getting started, for working things out, for getting more comfortable. It's for those who want a solid starting point, something concrete to work with.

If something resonates with you, if it seems useful, then great. If it doesn't that's great too because getting an idea of what doesn't work for you is important also.

If you are a new dominant who isn't sure yet what your dominance looks like exactly, if you're exploring, are perhaps a little unsure then this series of books is for you. If you are a new submissive trying to find your feet and struggling a little to get them firmly under you, this series of books is for you also.

Enjoy.
Sharyn Ferns

13 Easy Steps to Create an Amazing First Scene

So you're a new dominant and you've met a submissive who you really like and click with and you're heading into your very first ever play session. Yay!

You're probably scared shitless (it's okay, I won't tell). Nerves are normal: taking something that has lived in your head as a fantasy out into the real world with an honest-to-god real submissive partner is scary as hell. Trying to hang onto a 'dominant headspace', all confident and sure of yourself, can be really hard when the voice in your head is all fear and doubt.

This is the information I wish I'd had when I was a baby Domme and didn't have a clue what I was doing. I really wanted someone to just tell me 'how to do it right' and what I got instead was a lot of vague and non-specific advice that was no doubt correct, but not actually very helpful.

No-one wants to tell you what to do because there IS no 'right' or 'true' way, only what is right for you and of course everyone is different. I get that: It's 100%

true. But I wanted the 'how to' anyway just so I had some clue and wasn't floundering out there on my own.

So here it is. This guide gives you actionable steps to break down something that can be daunting into bite-sized, actionable pieces.

Before you start, if you're doing private play make sure you do all the work to get to know each other at least well enough that you both feel safe in a private space together. Negotiate limits and safewords and make sure you're both on the same page. None of this happens in a vacuum.

There is plenty of good information out there about safety (yours and theirs), negotiation, and consent: I'm not going to cover it here, that's not what this guide is for, so I'm going to assume you've done all that already (you have, right?!)*.

This guide is to give you some practical and actionable tips for planning your play, to give you a framework you can use so you have some direction, to give you something concrete that you can actually use.

BONUS: A free BDSM Scene Planner. The worksheet is a planning tool to help you implement the steps described in this guide to make your BDSM scene ah-mazing!

-//-

This guide does NOT explicitly walk through the details of safety, negotiation, or consent. If you are not familiar with those mandatory concepts, please ensure that you and your partner(s) get educated and are clear with each other well before you start planning any play. There are many great free resources available such as those found here:

https://www.domme-chronicles.com/link/kink-101.

1. Use a BDSM checklist

Talking about your interests is the first and best way to figure out what you want to include in your scene, but I know what it's like when you're new: You can get stuck at this first hurdle. You don't quite know what the options are, you may find that your submissive wants to leave everything up to you (protip: This doesn't work so well). A BDSM checklist is a great tool to get past this.

Both of you fill in a BDSM checklist separately if you haven't already.

You've probably heard of a BDSM checklist, maybe filled one out at some stage. A BDSM checklist generally has pages and pages (and pages and pages) of BDSM activities on it that you and your partner rate from NO (hard limit) to 5 (wild turn-on). The good checklists ask if you have done the activity before, and allow you to add notes.

If you don't have one, Google 'BDSM checklist' and you will find them: Best to grab one that is editable, check what it has on it, and add any specific things that you like that you want to get their take on (many checklists skew M/f, so if you have a male submissive and like cock rings or ball stretching or cross dressing, make sure they are on the list).

Alternatively, here is a link to an editable checklist that I use:

https://www.domme-chronicles.com/link/bdsm-checklist.

When you fill yours in try not to think about what your submissive likes or wants. This is about YOU. You will, of course, consider what your submissive likes and wants, but not now.

This seems like a good time to add that there are no inherently 'dominant' or 'submissive' acts and you don't need to be concerned about whether, say, having penis-in-vagina (PIV) sex suddenly makes you the submissive.

Think about it this way: If you want it, and you tell your submissive you want it, and you get it, that's pretty much the domliest dominance that ever dommed. And you don't have to dom-it-up by being extra bitchy or shouty or humiliating to make it so.

So forget all that noise and just think about things that are hot and fun for you, and mark them accordingly.

2. Pick favourite activities

Review your submissive's checklist alongside your own and note which ones you both scored as 'hell yes!'

Choose no more than 3 or 4 specific BDSM activities from the checklist as your 'main events'. Pick activities that you both marked as '5 – wild turn-on', your absolute favourites, and choose only things that you actually know how to do and will feel confident and safe doing.

What falls into that 'feel confident and safe' category may seem like 'not enough', too tame, not BDSM-ey enough. Let that feeling go. For real.

If you want to learn various skills with different implements, that's great! And if you want to learn them with (or on) this submissive, that's fine too. But having a learning experience with your submissive is a very different type of interaction from what we are aiming for here.

So only choose the 'feel confident and can do safely' things, there's still plenty. For example:

- light restraints with cuffs
- hand spanking
- tease and denial

- oral, giving

Whatever 3 or 4 things you choose will be the main blocks of your play: You will plan your time together around these things.

Also take note of the type of things that you both like even if they're not the focus of play.

By that I mean things like nudity, wearing cuffs, kneeling, slave positions, kissing, nipple torture, arse play, crawling etc. You can use that information even if you aren't specifically making the play about that. For example, if crawling is something that's on both of your 'yes please' lists then you know that it's okay to have them crawl from one room to another, even if that's not your focus this time.

3. WRITE A LITTLE EROTIC STORY

Relax somewhere quiet and visualise how you see the play going using those things you've identified.

You've probably done this in your head plenty of times, but this time it has to be realistic and detailed (how do you start, what do you want them to wear, what is the mood like, how do you talk to them, what do you want from them, how do you ask for those things, how do you move from one activity to the next, how will you check in with them, how do you finish the session, etc.).

Write it down.

That forces you to think about actual for-real practicalities like 'oh, I guess I can't hang from that beam and shoot lasers at their arse BECAUSE I DON'T HAVE A LASER GUN' etc.

Don't make yourself (or them) into a totally different person in your story. If you are cuddly and sweet, don't change your entire personality into 'Mistress Bitchy Pants' for this. It's great to stretch your comfort zone some, and it can be fun to role play, but don't put too much pressure on yourself. You aren't putting on a stage performance, you are exploring what makes you and your partner feel good.

If your story is not super-hot-awesome-fun for you, start again. It should make you excited.

The story will have things in it that you didn't list in the previous step because once you play it out in your head, you will think of things you want to do that you didn't consider. Double check that everything in your story is on the 'okay' list for your submissive.

While the 3-4 main activities should be on both of your '5 - wild turn-on' list, not everything has to be a 5. So if, say, crawling is listed as a 3 or 4 as in 'yeah, that's okay' for them, then as long as the play isn't all about crawling, include it if you want.

Do not for one second imagine that things will go the way they do in your story: This isn't a movie and you haven't created a script for players to follow. That's not how life works.

This exercise is to fire you up and give you ideas, to see for yourself what you are trying to create (not just the acts, but the feelings, the interactions, the exchange between you and your submissive).

If you have a sexual relationship by all means include all the 'vanilla' sexy things in your story. Don't be concerned that it's 'too vanilla' so it doesn't count somehow. You want it? You can have it (with consent and within your agreed limits of course). This is one of the great joys of being the dominant.

You can use this kind of exercise to learn what you want your play to look and feel like and to explicitly figure out what activities light you up.

4. Make a Playlist

From the little story make a list of things you want to do in the order you want to do them.

Then check that everything on your list is a '3 or above' on your submissive's checklist. If it's not, pull it out. This is not because you can never do things that aren't their favourite or because you're pandering, it's because for your first BDSM scene, you will gain confidence by choosing activities that you will both love and that have the highest likelihood of creating something amazing for both of you.

Your playlist is not a script, but you can take the list into the playroom with you to use as a prompt if you want to. You may not need it, and you certainly don't have to stick to it, but it's a nice little backup if you get flustered.

Tease your submissive with things that are on the playlist: This both builds anticipation and also acts as a check that they are excited about those things.

If you have any doubt about their enthusiasm, actually give them a list of possible activities for your play time and literally get them to say an enthusiastic 'yes!' to everything on it. This kind of explicit communication can reinforce your choices, give you up-front consent (with awareness that when they are in the middle of it, they might change their minds and that's okay), and bolster your confidence in knowing that they are excited to do those things with you.

Be clear with them (if you show them) and with yourself (for your own peace of mind) that this is NOT a 'will do' list: This is really important. The playlist is not some contract where you are committing to doing all of those things. Depending how play goes, you may not. So set expectations that this is a 'might possibly maybe do' list of ideas.

Note: *I mentioned at the start of this guide that I am not explicitly covering negotiation or safety or consent as separate topics in this guide, but to be clear: What I'm describing here assumes that all of this is happening in the context of negotiated boundaries and limits, and assumes that you both have a clear understanding of enthusiastic consent before, during and after play. If that's not the case, go get on that.*

5. USE A BLINDFOLD

A blindfold can be both hot and disorientating for them, and a confidence boost for you.

If you are nervous, it hides those nerves very well and it's nice to know that if you do get flustered they won't see you faffing about or checking the playlist or fumbling with things while you figure out what to do next.

A blindfold can be like a security blanket, so if it's on both of your checklists as a '3 or above', use one.

Seriously, it's great.

6. FAKE IT 'TIL YOU MAKE IT

If you don't feel confident, act it.

In the lead up and during play behave in a way that supports that feeling. I don't mean be some blustery-bluster chest beating cliché or pretend that you are all-knowing and all-powerful: That's just lying.

I mean find your voice and your stride and practice projecting them even if you are a little tremulous inside. It may seem strange, but outwardly confident presentation and external validation of it helps to bolster confidence.

Literally practice your voice. Practice speaking as if you expect to be obeyed. It doesn't have to be loud and barky (though, you know, if that's your thing go for it), it just has to be a voice that shows authority.

It often doesn't come naturally, so it can help to practice it. If it helps, I sometimes think of it as my 'dog voice'. Ever had a dog? You don't equivocate with dogs. If you want your dog to sit, you look at them, you point to the floor, and you tell them clearly and firmly: "Sit". And they do. Yeah, use that voice.

Give your submissive some instructions prior to play time. It may be random small things in the days leading up to it, it may be about what to wear for you on the day, or work they can do to help set up the space beforehand. It doesn't have to be anything huge. The point is not the thing you are asking for, the point is having some practice asserting yourself and your submissive having some practice doing what you say. Also it's fun. And hot.

Do some self-talk that affirms your own amazingness (is SO a word!). I know that sounds airy fairy and I'm not that person, but according to plenty of psychological studies, self-talk can be effective. As an example: "I am strong, I am powerful, I am dominant. This is who I am."

Revel in the fact that someone likes and trusts you enough to do this with you. If you and your submissive are that way inclined, have them write you some kind of tribute to your awesomeness. Perhaps give them a question prompt: "What is it about me that makes you want to submit to me?"

Believe your submissive when they give you 'that' look, when they say 'those' words: They already know you're all that, you just have to believe it yourself, or at least, act as if you do until you internalise that truth.

7. PREPARE YOURSELF AND YOUR SPACE

Set up your play space to your liking: candles, lighting, music, whatever suits your mood and style.

Walk through your playlist from Step 4 in your head and get everything you plan to use out and have it to hand in the relevant spot so you don't have to go searching for 'stuff' once you get started. It's not only for play-readiness, but to set the mood for you.

Planning on restraining them? How? Get cuffs out, put ropes around the bed, attach the clips already, so all you have to do is clip the cuffs in.

Planning on teasing? What with? Have feathers, toys, lube ready.

Put out the blindfold if you're using one.

Need wipes?

A towel?

Some custard?

Have all of that within easy reach.

Do all the grooming that makes you feel pampered and fresh and fabulous. Put on your favourite scent.

Shave or wax whatever bits you prefer to be hairless (or none, if that's not your thing).

Wear something that makes you feel 'raawwwrrrr' level of awesome-powerful. Doesn't matter what it is.

You want to go full uber-domly domdom with some amazing leather and latex number and the full shebang? Do that. You want to wear sweat pants and your favourite t-shirt? Great. Nudity is your thing? Go for it.

8. TAKE THINGS SLOW

Going slowly builds tension and it allows you the space and time to build up your confidence.

When we are full of nervous energy we often rush and run about, so if you find yourself doing that, consciously take some deep breaths and try and think about moving and speaking with thoughtful deliberation.

Don't be afraid of silence or stillness, even if it's because you're not sure what to do next. As far as your submissive is concerned, it's your choice to be silent or still, and usually that makes them really nervous wondering what you are up to, which is just hot.

There is no hurry, so if you feel yourself start to get a bit frantic or flustered, just stop, take a deep breath, and relax for a moment. Your submissive isn't going anywhere.

9. KEEP IT SHORT

Don't try and create some huge ten-act operatic performance out of it.

When you get experienced and comfortable with yourself and with them, you may have play sessions that last for hours and hours, and that's great. But for the first one, plan to keep it short so that you don't feel like you're under any pressure.

Let them know up-front that you are only giving them a taster, feeling them out. That sets expectations.

Better to end on an 'aw, too soon' high than have it peter out because you ran out of steam or ideas.

If, after doing all of these steps, you end up with a playlist that looks daunting to you, cut it down to something that feels fun and manageable.

The best outcome is that this first-time play leaves you both (really really) wanting more.

10. CHECK IN OFTEN

If you have an experienced submissive, you have a great resource in them: Use it. Ask them before you play how they react to different sensations so you have more information. Talk to them about how they like to communicate during play.

If they are not experienced then you will have to work a little harder because even if you discuss safewords and in-play communication with them, they may find themselves incapable of logical thought in the midst of it.

During play watch your submissive's reactions carefully.

Are they arching up for more, are they flinching to get away, are they stoically still, are they moaning, crying, silent? Are they suddenly reacting differently than before?

While you can often tell what different reactions mean, when you are new and it's the first time you've played with this person, even if you pay attention, reactions can be hard to interpret.

If you are unsure, ask.

And I don't care if you kill your submissive's buzz. Truly, I don't. Because you have to keep them safe and you have to keep yourself safe, and if doing that is a bummer for them, they can just get over it.

The 'big boots stomping over everything' image of the domly domdomdom might be hot, but in reality, it's a recipe for disaster. When you know yourself and them well, THEN bring in the big boots and stomp away. First time play with a new partner is not the time.

Sometimes you ARE sure where they are in the moment because it's bleeding obvious, and it's easy. But until you know your partner and their reactions really well, better to check in too much than not enough. It doesn't have to be mood-killing:

"You doing okay there, baby?"

"Do you want some more?"

"Tell me where you're at: scale of 1-10." *[obviously work out the scale beforehand: pleasure, pain, etc.]*

"Tell me how many more you want/can take."

"If you want more, beg me for it..."

Keep in mind here that most submissives want to please their dominant, so pay attention not just to what they say, but how they say it. Ask them several times if you want more of a chance to gauge what they mean, "Are you sure? Really sure? Then ask me for it" or something similar. A reluctant 'yes I want some more' is a no.

Err on the side of caution, always.

You can back out of an activity with an assertion of your own if you think they might feel bad for stopping you (they shouldn't, ever, but human nature is what it is). Try something like "No, you don't deserve any more of that" or "No, I'm going to move onto something else now" if you want to make it seem like it's simply your decision. Talk about any ambiguities afterwards and re-calibrate for next time if you misread it.

It is always **always** ALWAYS much better to leave your submissive wanting more than to find out after the fact that you went too far.

11. IF SOMETHING ISN'T WORKING, STOP IT

Sometimes things just... don't work.

People don't talk about this enough because it's not sexy, but it's true.

In all the fantasies every single thing is hot as hell and every touch is orgasmic and every sigh is one of endless pleasure and delight. But if you think back to all of the sexual interactions you've had, there have been awkward moments, apologies as you smash your elbow into someone's face, when you get a bit bored with something, etc. It happens.

BDSM play is no different.

It doesn't matter how experienced you are; the first time you play with someone, you just don't know how they're going to react to different activities. And if you are new, you probably don't know how *you* are going to react either. Things that seem hot and fun in fantasy may actually fall flat. It's not anyone's fault, it just happens sometimes.

Let me repeat that: IT'S NOT ANYONE'S FAULT.

And when I say 'doesn't work', there is a wide range of what that might look like. The easiest way to describe it is to say that you feel nothing: no enjoyment, no excitement, no curiosity, no fun, no energy return from your submissive, it just feels like you are in some kind of 'dead space' even though you are actively doing something.

So if you aren't feeling good about how an activity is going, what can you do?

You can try and change it up a little bit to see if you can make it work. Sometimes you can push through that feeling and come up with something amazing on the other side, so do give it a go.

For example, if you are doing some impact play, you can try alternating it with gentle touches. If you are doing some teasing, you can make them tell you how it feels. Feel free to play around with it to try and see if you can find something that sparkles.

But if continuing with that activity is starting to sap your confidence because it doesn't feel right, don't keep trying to beat a dead horse. Wind it down and move on.

Your playlist can be helpful here, just take a breath, and go on to the next thing you had planned.

Don't apologise, don't panic, don't make a big deal out of it, just move on. You can discuss it afterwards to see how it felt to your submissive (sometimes you might be surprised that they didn't even notice anything was wrong).

And the ultimate 'if something isn't working' is if *nothing* you try is working. Nobody talks about this either, but sometimes there is simply a mismatch in play styles or expectations and you can't get the play off the ground at all. For example, if you are a reaction junkie like me, and you are with a play partner who is stoic and still, that's always going to be a struggle and it may simply be a compatibility problem that you may not realise until you try.

If for some reason you aren't getting anything out of it, or it seems like they aren't getting anything out of it, if it just feels 'off' all round, it's okay to wind the entire scene down, end it, and resolve to have a chat about it later (not immediately afterwards: you will probably both be feeling a little fragile, so best to just be sweet with each other and suggest that you talk about it in more detail later).

It will be disappointing for you and it will be disappointing for them, but after a certain point, it's better to stop than it is to 'soldier on' hoping it will get better. If YOU aren't feeling it, then it's unlikely that they will feel it, and trying to force it is probably going to make you feel worse.

And if it does fall flat, be gentle with them and, perhaps even more importantly, be gentle with yourself. Sometimes learning new things is hard and sometimes it won't go so well and THAT'S OKAY. Seriously.

There is a learning curve here, and how steep it is depends on a lot of factors so be kind to yourself if things don't go exactly as you had hoped.

-//-

On a related note, if you're a new dominant, you may have an expectation that physical signs of your submissive's arousal will be at 100% throughout, for example that their cock is going to be hard the entire time you are playing (frankly, new subs may have that expectation also). That belief can lead you to focus on their physical excitement as confirmation that you're 'doing it right', and get into a kind of panic if that's not the case (if we're talking cocks, that voice in your head might start yelling 'Oh hell, their cock's not hard, that means they aren't enjoying this and I'm a huge faaaaiiillluuurrreee WHAT CAN I DO TO MAKE THEIR COCK HARD AGAIN??!!111').

Your submissive's physical arousal is not a barometer by which to measure your 'success' as a dominant or to measure how well the play is going.

Many factors influence how bodies react: The individual's natural response, the type of play, fear level, nerves, how they process sensations, how much pain is involved, how much they're concentrating, etc.

It's perfectly normal for physical arousal to wax and wane, and if it wanes, that doesn't mean they aren't enjoying it. In fact it might mean that their senses are so joyously overloaded that their genitals have become irrelevant while they revel in what is going on.

If you aren't sure that they are having a good time, check in with them (but be careful not to implicitly or explicitly pressure them with your expectations). Trust them if they say they are enjoying it.

12. STARTING AND ENDING RITUAL

A ritual can be a shortcut into a D/s mindset, so it can be useful to clearly signal 'starting now' and 'ending now' vs kind of 'sliding into it' which can be unclear and messy.

So signal the start cleanly.

One idea is to have them kneel in a position that is hot for you, and maybe have them affirm their submission to you by repeating some mantra. Or inspect their body, comment on how pretty they are, give them hints of what you are going to have them do.

Have a think about something that makes you think 'ooh, YES!'

It can be useful to remind them of their safewords at this point (commonly yellow for 'hold on I need a word' and red for 'everything stops now'). It's a good reminder of their responsibility in play to let you know if something isn't right.

You don't have to put on a stern voice or be anyone other than yourself as you go through the starting ritual. Do what feels right, sexy, hot to you. They will feed off your energy.

Signal the end cleanly when you are done.

At the end, wind down slowly vs having a hard stop (that is, slow down whatever you are doing, perhaps some gentle touching vs just suddenly moving away and declaring 'done now!'). Then it can be useful to have a ritual that signals that you are ending the scene.

Perhaps the reverse of the starting ritual.

You could have them kneel, take off their cuffs, gently touch and comment on marks if there are any, some literal petting, telling them what a good boy/girl/pet they were for you, how well they did, how proud you are of them, etc.

Take the opportunity to segue into whatever aftercare you have agreed on.

13. AFTERCARE

When you are new, or if your submissive is new, you may not yet know if you need aftercare or what kind of aftercare you need, but be aware that either or both of you may well need it.

Search the internet for information on sub-drop and top-drop/dom-drop and talk to your submissive about this up-front. Many dominants suffer from drop, so even if your sub is experienced and says that they don't need aftercare, negotiate it for yourself in case *you* need it.

Even if you don't play very hard, BDSM can have unexpected emotional and physical impacts for both parties, and especially if this is the first time you have played, the feelings afterwards can be very confusing.

For both play partners: Your body may release endorphins and adrenaline when you play, and as they dissipate you may feel depressed, sad, listless as you come down. Or you may feel shame or guilt afterwards, you may worry that there's something wrong with you, you may need reassurance that you're still a good person and that they still like you, you may feel lonely or scared that you crossed a line.

A whole mess of bad or unexpected feels might sneak up on you in the hours or days afterwards. Your submissive might feel the same.

Personally I can drop like a stone after play and I need lots of affection and togetherness and warmth from my submissive to short circuit it: Often that's the kind of aftercare that has worked for my submissive also, so it feeds us both. But everyone is different.

At a minimum, have some protein and snacks (chocolate, nuts, protein bars) and water available for afterwards, and ensure that you plan some time together immediately after you play. Physical contact can help, whether it's cuddles or having them kneel at your feet so you can pet them. Keep in touch in the day or two that follow even if it's just a text or two to check in: It's not only polite and reassuring, but knowing that your sub is okay is part of your responsibility. Plus if you are dropping yourself, having that contact can help.

So even if you think that sounds unlikely, be aware of it, negotiate the 'just in case' scenario for both of you. And don't think that because you are the dominant, you are somehow immune to it.

Yes, you have to care for your submissive afterwards, but they need to care for you also.

A Worked Example

Here's an example of what it might look like for me if
followed the tips (the bold items expanded below).

1. Use a BDSM checklist
2. **Pick activities that are favourites for both of you**
3. **Write a little erotic story that includes those things**
4. **Make a playlist based on the story**
5. **Fake it 'til you make it.**
6. **Prepare yourself and your environment**
7. **Have a starting and ending ritual**
8. Use a blindfold
9. Take things slow
10. If something isn't working, stop doing it
11. **Check in with your submissive often**
12. Keep it short
13. Aftercare

-//-

2. **Pick activities** *[from the BDSM checklist]* **that are favourites for both of you**
   Main Activities *(the 3-4 favourites, the focus of play)*:
   Being restrained
   Tease & denial
   Hand spanking
   Other *(all things that are good with him that I might use)*:
   Nudity, body inspection, collar/cuffs/leash, blindfold, kneeling, crawling, kissing, biting, nipple play, pinching, face sitting, hand jobs (giving/receiving).

3. **Write a little erotic story that includes those things**
   I greet him at the door, dressed in my blue strappy summer dress and my favourite heels, even though heels are entirely inappropriate for wearing at home. I invite him in, point to the middle of the living room.
   "Stand there," I say.
   He does. He waits.
   I take a seat on the couch, take my time looking at him.
   "Take off your clothes."

He starts undressing, quickly undoing buttons while trying to get his shoes off.

"No. Slowly." I watch him.

When he is finally naked, I have him fold his clothes, place them on the edge of the couch.

I get up then and walk around him, touching him gently.

I whisper in his hear, "Hands behind your head."

He complies and I examine him like he is a prized animal. Grabbing, pinching, stroking. I make him open his mouth and touch his tongue, his teeth.

When I am happy that I have looked over every inch of him, I go back to my seat on the couch, reach for the cuffs. He stays put, watching me.

I snap my fingers and point to the floor at my feet. He hurries to kneel before me.

I open a wrist cuff and hold it open towards him. He gently places his wrist against the leather and I tighten it on him and do up the buckle. We repeat this on his other wrist.

I hold the collar towards him and he lowers his head towards my knees until his forehead is on my thighs. I close the collar around his neck and check that it's comfortable.

Then I lift his head by the chin, pick up the leash, and clip it onto the D-ring at the front of the collar. I smile and give it a little tug. He looks up at me.

"It suits you," I say.

He smiles back, nods. "Yes, Ma'am."

"What are you here for?" I ask.

He gives me the answer I have had him learn, "I'm here to please you, Ma'am."

"Tell me what you want."

"I want to submit to you, Ma'am."

I nod my approval. "Then crawl for me."

I stand up and start slowly towards the bedroom, the leash in my hand. He follows close behind, naked and on all fours.

...

[I'm not going to write out the entire thing, I think you get the idea]

4. Make a playlist based on the story

- Strip, hands behind head, body inspection
- Kneeling, cuffs, collar on
- Crawling on leash to bedroom, wait in the corner
- Blindfold
- Attached face-up to the bed, crawl all over him, teasing, biting
- Kissing, offering body parts to his mouth for kisses

- Nipple play, check-in for intensity
- Facesit tease, but no
- Release clips, re-attach face down
- Arse spanking, light to heavier, check-ins
- Tell him to lift his arse, teasing
- Let him feel my pussy
- Decide if he gets to come and/or if he gets to make me come
- Release clips
- Wind down: petting, whispering, kissing, cuddling
- Have him kneel, take off collar, cuffs, say 'thank you' to me
- Pour out all the sweetness
- Aftercare

5. Fake it 'til you make it

Have a short session where we just practice him going to his knees until he can do it elegantly.

Tell him I expect him to comply when I say 'kneel': Practice that at random times (so hot!).

Hone the above so that when I snap my fingers and point to the ground he will kneel.

Practice the starting ritual exchange:

"What are you here for?"

"I'm here to please you, Ma'am."

"Tell me what you want."

"I want to submit to you, Ma'am."

Tell him to get aftercare snacks.

Have him model the kind of underwear that I like so I can choose one for him to wear.

Make a list of things that HE can do to get the space ready for our scene and give that to him.

Tell him to address me as 'Ma'am' in every sentence for an afternoon so he gets used to it.

Tell him to write me 500 words on what he hopes to get out of our scene.

6. Prepare yourself and your environment

Put ropes on the bed with clips.

Put cuffs, collar, and leash in the living room.

Put blindfold, lube, flogger, crop on the bedside table.

Draw bedroom curtains, make room temperature comfortable.

Put on lacy lingerie under a pretty summer dress, favourite heels. Do hair and makeup.

Get nuts, chocolate, water for aftercare.

7. Have a starting and ending ritual

Starting: Stand silently in the centre of the room, submit to body inspection.

Ending: Kneel, take off collar and cuffs, have him say 'Thank you, Ma'am'.

11. Check in with your submissive often

Phrases to use:

- Are you doing okay there, baby?
- Do you want some more of this? Tell me.
- Do you like that, boy?
- How many more do you want?

BONUS: FREE BDSM SCENE PLANNER

This BDSM scene planner is based on the principles described in this book. It will help you plan and run your play session by implementing the steps you've just read about.

Below is a preview of the four page planner which you can download here:

https://www.domme-chronicles.com/link/bdsm-scene-planner

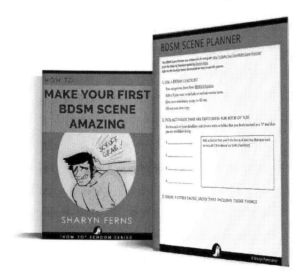

So, What Now?

This may seem daunting at first, but when you gain some more skills and experience, when you grow your confidence, you will relax into your dominance, find your own style, learn what you love.

All of this is just a set of tools, none of it is mandatory or sanctioned by some 'Domly Board of How To Do Things'. It's a springboard, that's all. A firm footing if you need it. If you find any of it useful, that's great. If you don't, that's great too. It means you've learnt what *doesn't* work for you.

I do want to say this because it's important: Many new dominant women concentrate their play on 'blowing their submissive's mind'. There is *nothing* wrong with that, it's awesome, and it feels powerful, and this guide will work well to facilitate that. And if you love that, you go!

But don't lose sight of your own desires.

If you lose hold of your own pleasure, you can start to feel like you are doing a bunch of work to pander to your submissive and that's not sustainable. You may [both] start measuring your 'dominance' by how pleased your submissive is with your 'performance' as a dominant. But your dominance is not a performance acted out for his approval. That will end up making you get burnt out and it can start to feel like the opposite of dominance. You may start to wonder 'what's in it for me?'

So if it feels exhausting over time, as if you are doing all of the giving and getting nothing back, if your submissive is looking to you to continually 'do for them' and it's not feeling right or powerful or sexy to you, then don't be afraid to stop and think about it.

It doesn't mean you aren't 'dominant enough', it doesn't mean D/s isn't for you. It just means you have to take a breather and look at what's going on. Ask yourself what *you* want. Maybe you just haven't found your rhythm yet. Or perhaps you haven't found the right submissive yet.

Don't be afraid to say that something isn't working for you. Making a relationship and play work is not somehow solely down to you because you're the dominant: You and your submissive are in this together. You are creating this play and this relationship as a team, and you both need to be active participants in making it successful.

You are a fabulous dominant woman who deserves the kind of play and relationship that you love, and if you doubt it, go look in the mirror and have a word with yourself :).

In the end, do what feels right for you and your partner, make it safe and hot and intense and awesome.

And most of all, have fun with it.

About the Author

Sharyn Ferns is an experienced dominant woman who started her BDSM explorations over 20 years ago. She has been writing the award-winning Domme Chronicles blog for more than eight years, and moderates an F/m discussion group of some 80,000 members. This 'How To' Femdom series is born out of her experiences and the interactions and conversations she has been having with dominant women and submissive men over those many years.

She is passionate about submissive men, about writing, creative thinking, mindful living, and about seeing beauty in the world. She's a confirmed introvert despite the fact that she spews every intimate detail of her personal life out in public with verve and enthusiasm.

As a dominant, she is loving and selfish, affectionate and demanding, generous and uncompromising, deeply passionate and reserved. Complex and unique, like most people.

-//-

Other books in this 'How To' Femdom series include:

- How To Write An Awesome Online Profile
- How To Find A Dominant Woman
- More to come

To be the first to hear about new book releases, sign up to her mailing list:

https://www.domme-chronicles.com/link/mailing-list

-//-

She is known as 'Ferns' online, and you can connect with her at:

Books: https://books.domme-chronicles.com

W: https://www.domme-chronicles.com

T: @Ferns___ (double underscore!)

F: https://www.facebook.com/Ferns.DommeChronicles

FL: https://fetlife.com/Ferns

E: ferns@domme-chronicles.com

-//-

If you found this guide useful, please consider writing a short Amazon review: As an independent author, word-of-mouth is key, and reviews really help other readers to find my books.

Made in the USA
Coppell, TX
27 December 2019

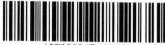

13798084R00032